Step-By-Step Obesity Remedy:

A Complete Guide to Overcome Obesity and Living a Healthier Life

By 

Henry K. Chestnut

Table Of Content

Step-by-step obesity remedy

Introduction

Understanding Obesity

Obesity is a complex and prevalent health issue that has become a global epidemic over the past few decades. It is characterized by an excessive accumulation of body fat, which can have detrimental effects on an individual's health and well-being. This problem is not limited to a specific age group, gender, or geographical location; it affects people of all backgrounds and has significant social, economic, and medical implications.

Understanding obesity, its causes, consequences, and potential solutions is crucial for individuals, healthcare professionals, and society as a whole.

Understanding obesity

Obesity is more than just an aesthetic concern; it is a multifaceted health condition with numerous contributing factors. While the primary cause of obesity is an imbalance between calories consumed and calories expended, several interconnected elements play a role in its development. These factors include genetic predisposition, environmental influences, lifestyle choices, and socioeconomic factors.

Some Key components of understanding obesity include:

Body Mass Index (BMI): BMI is a widely used measure to classify individuals as underweight, normal weight, overweight, or obese. It is a person's weight in kilograms (or pounds) divided by the square of their height in meters (or feet).

Health consequences

Obesity is associated with a higher risk of various health issues, including heart disease, type 2 diabetes, hypertension, certain cancers, and musculoskeletal disorders. It can also lead to mental health concerns, such as depression and low self-esteem.

Causes of Obesity

Diet: Eating too many high-calorie, low-nutrient items, such as processed snacks, sugary drinks, and fast food, can lead to poor dietary choices and weight gain.

Physical Activity: Obesity and weight gain can result from a sedentary lifestyle with little exercise. The body burns fewer calories when it is not regularly exercised.

Emotional eating: Eating to relieve stress, emotions, and boredom can lead to obesity. Emotional eating is caused by stress, worry, and unhappiness.

Genetics: Obesity may be influenced by genetics. Some people may have a slower metabolism or be genetically inclined to gaining weight more quickly. Genetics, however, is not the sole determinant; lifestyle decisions are also quite important.

Environment: A person's diet and exercise habits can be greatly influenced by the environment in which they reside. Obesity rates can be influenced by socioeconomic variables, safe locations for physical activity, and access to healthful food.

Socioeconomic status: Due to limited access to wholesome meals, healthcare, and opportunities for physical activity, those with lower incomes and education levels may be more likely to become obese.

Psychological variables: Stress, depression, or a history of trauma are examples of emotional and psychological variables that can cause overeating or bad eating habits, which in turn can contribute to obesity.

Medication: Obesity is a side effect of some drugs, including corticosteroids, antipsychotics, and some antidepressants.

Hormonal factors: Imbalances in hormones can have an impact on controlling weight. Weight gain can result from diseases such as hypothyroidism and polycystic ovarian syndrome (PCOS).

Sleep: Hormones that control hunger can be upset by getting too little or poor quality sleep, which can result in weight gain.

Childhood habits: Childhood habits have an impact on an adult's weight. Obesity is more frequent in children who have poor diet and activity habits.

Food marketing and advertising
Widespread marketing of unhealthy foods, particularly to children, has the potential to impact food choices and lead to overconsumption of calorie-dense, low-nutrient options.

Social and psychological aspects of obesity

Obesity can lead to social stigma and discrimination, affecting a person's quality of life and mental health. Understanding the social and psychological impact of obesity is essential for addressing the condition holistically.

The importance of addressing obesity

Addressing obesity is of paramount importance for several reasons:

Health and Well-Being: Obesity is a major risk factor for a range of chronic diseases and conditions. Addressing obesity can significantly improve an individual's health and overall well-being, reducing the burden on healthcare systems.

Economic impact: The economic cost of obesity is substantial. Healthcare expenses related to obesity, as well as decreased work productivity, impose a heavy financial burden on individuals and society.

Quality of life: Obesity can limit mobility, decrease life expectancy, and diminish the quality of life. By addressing obesity, people can enjoy a better quality of life and increased longevity.

Prevention: Preventing obesity is more effective and cost-efficient than treating it once it has developed. Promoting healthier lifestyles and environments can help prevent obesity in the first place.

Social equality: Addressing obesity is essential to reducing health disparities, as it disproportionately affects marginalized and underserved populations. Promoting equity in healthcare and access to nutritious food is crucial.

Understanding Obesity-Related Health Risks

Numerous hazards and problems for one's health are linked to obesity. Understanding the major health effects of obesity requires awareness of these hazards. Among the most prevalent health hazards associated with obesity are:

(a) **Type 2 Diabetes**: One of the main risk factors for type 2 diabetes is obesity. Insulin resistance, which is brought on by excess body fat, makes it more difficult for the body to control blood sugar levels.

(b) **Cardiovascular disease**: Being obese raises your risk of developing heart disease as well as disorders that are linked to it, such as high blood pressure, atherosclerosis, and stroke.

(c) **Hypertension**: An abundance of adipose tissue can cause hypertension, which puts stress on the heart and blood vessels and raises the risk of heart disease. low levels of HDL cholesterol and high levels of triglycerides and LDL cholesterol. This makes atherosclerosis worse.

(d) **Respiratory Issue**: Obesity can result in breathing issues, including sleep apnea, which lowers oxygen intake and causes poor sleep quality.

(e) **Osteoarthritis:** Carrying more weight strains joints, especially the hips and knees, which can result in osteoarthritis and persistent joint discomfort.

(f) **Fatty Liver Disease:** NAFLD, or Non-Alcoholic Fatty Liver Disease, is more prevalent in obese individuals and has the potential to worsen liver disorders.

(g) **Gastroesophageal Reflux Disease (GERD):** Obesity might raise the risk of GERD, which can result in persistent acid reflux and other digestive issues.

(h) **Certain Cancers**: Breast, colorectal, and endometrial cancers are among the cancers that are linked to an increased risk of obesity.

(i) **Stroke:** Obesity increases the risk of stroke, especially when combined with other cardiovascular risk factors, including hypertension.

(j) **Sleep Disorders**: Insomnia and sleep apnea, two conditions that can negatively affect general health and quality of life, are associated with obesity.

(k) **Mental Health Problems:** Individuals who are obese may experience stigma, discrimination, and mental health problems like depression and low self-esteem.

(l) **Infertility:** Hormonal abnormalities and infertility in men and women can be caused by obesity.

(m) **Pregnancy complications:** Women who are obese during pregnancy are more likely to experience gestational diabetes, preeclampsia, and difficulties giving birth.

(n) **Diminished life expectancy**: Because obesity raises the risk of these and other illnesses, it is generally linked to a lower life expectancy.

(o) **Family and personal health history**: Consider your family's history of obesity and related health conditions. Reflect on your personal medical history to identify any obesity-related issues you may already be facing.

Chapter 1

Assessing Your Current Situation

Assessing your existing position is an important initial step in any self-improvement process, including efforts to address issues such as weight management, health, or personal well-being. This evaluation will help you obtain insight on where you stand, identify areas of concern, and chart a course for your journey. Here's how to examine your current condition effectively:

(a) **Self-reflection**: Begin by devoting some time to self-reflection.

(b) Ask yourself important questions about your current health, lifestyle, and well-being. Consider your weight, eating habits, physical activity, sleep patterns, and emotional state. Be honest with yourself about your strengths and opportunities for improvement. Consider arranging a health check-up with a healthcare provider. This can include metrics such as your weight, body mass index (BMI), blood pressure, cholesterol levels and blood sugar levels are both important. Discuss your overall health as well as any concerns you have.

(c) Goals and aspirations: Consider your personal goals and dreams. What goals do you have for your health and well-being? Are you seeking for particular weight loss objectives, or are you looking for a more general sense of increased health and vitality?

(d) Dietary evaluation: Examine your present eating habits. For a few days, keep a food journal to detail what you eat and drink. Take note of your portion quantities, meal times, and food types. This might provide information about your nutritional choices.

(e) **Physical activity**: Assess your degree of physical activity. Consider how frequently you exercise or engage in physical activity. Examine your physical condition. Evaluate your fitness level as well as any restrictions or barriers to staying active.

(f) **Sleep patterns**: Consider your sleep patterns and sleep quality. How long do you sleep at night? Do you have any sleep disorders, such as insomnia or sleep apnea?

(g) Stress and emotional well-being: Examine your stress and emotional well-being levels.

Determine your causes of stress and how you currently deal with them. Are you prone to emotional eating or other stress-related behaviors?

(h) System of support: Consider the level of accountability and support in your life. Do you have any friends, family, or support networks who can aid you along the way? Consider your own motivation and determination.

(i)   **Medical issues:** Consider any current medical issues or health concerns you may have. These can make a big difference in your weight management and overall health.

(j)   **Psychological evaluation**: Consider your thoughts and attitude toward change. Are you ready and motivated to make changes in your life to improve your health and well-being?

Your weight and body mass index (BMI)

Understanding Body Weight: Begin by stepping on a scale to measure your current body weight. Note that weight alone is not a complete indicator of your health. It's crucial to assess your overall well-being.

How to calculating your BMI

BMI is a useful tool to estimate whether your weight falls within a healthy range. Calculate your BMI by dividing your weight in kilograms by your height in meters squared (BMI = weight (kg) / (height (m) * height (m)).

Use BMI categories to understand where you stand:

Underweight: BMI less than 18.5

Normal weight: BMI 18.5 to 24.9

Overweight: BMI 25 to 29.9

Obese: BMI 30 or greater

Chapter 2

Designing a Weight Loss Plan

In your journey to lose weight, it's essential to create a comprehensive plan that takes into consideration various factors. Below are the tips for choosing the right approach, setting a realistic timeline, and consulting with a healthcare professional.

(a) Diet plan

Your diet plays an important role in your weight-loss process. The following factors should be considered when choosing a diet plan:

Caloric Reduction: Weight loss typically requires a reduction in calorie consumption. Calculate your daily caloric needs and create a caloric deficit for gradual and sustainable weight loss.

Nutrient-rich foods: Focus on whole, nutrient-dense foods such as fruits, vegetables, lean proteins, and whole grains. Minimize processed and high-sugar foods.

Control portion: Be conscious of the size of food you eat to avoid eating less or more, even with healthy foods.

Hydration: Drinking plenty of water can help control hunger and support metabolism.

Meal Planning: Plan your meals appropriately and avoid unhealthy choices.

(b). Exercise

Incorporating physical activity into your weight loss plan is essential for overall health and improved results. Consider the following:

Cardiovascular exercise: Activities such as walking, jogging, cycling, or swimming help burn calories and improve cardiovascular health.

Strength training: Building muscle can increase your metabolism and help with long-term weight control and management.

Consistency: Establish a regular exercise routine that you can maintain over time.

Variety: Mix different types of exercises to prevent boredom and work different muscle groups.

Consult a trainer: If you're new to exercise, consider working with a fitness trainer to ensure you're using proper techniques.

(c) Behavioral changes

Changing your habits and behaviors is crucial for successful, sustainable weight loss. Here are some behavioral aspects to consider:

Intuitive eating: Pay key attention to what and when you eat, and let your body guide you in making food choices.

Manage stress: Avoid high-stress levels to prevent serious health problems like obesity, high blood pressure, and depression. Find healthy ways to balance stress, like meditation or yoga.

Lifestyle adjustments: Focus on creating long-term, healthy habits rather than rushing to meet a specific deadline.

(d) Setting realistic weight loss goals

Realistic goals are essential for long-term success. Setting achievable targets helps maintain motivation and reduces the risk of disappointment.

Consult a healthcare professional: Before setting weight-loss goals, consult a healthcare professional or a registered dietitian.

They can provide personalized advice and ensure your goals are safe and appropriate for your unique situation.

Establishing specific goals: Your weight-loss goals should be specific, measurable, and time-bound.

Gradual and sustainable changes: Focus on making gradual, attainable changes to your diet and physical activity. Avoid extreme diets or physical activity regimens that are difficult to maintain.

Goal setting: Set clear and achievable goals for your weight-loss journey.

Accountability: Consider sharing your goals with a friend or joining a support group to stay accountable.

Tracking progress: Use a weight-loss application or a journal to monitor your food intake, exercise, and make adjustments when necessary.

Plateaus: Be prepared for periods where your weight may temporarily stabilize or even increase despite your efforts. This is expected and should not discourage you from continuing the process.

Planning healthy eating habits

In your quest for effective weight management and overall well-being, developing healthy eating habits is paramount. This chapter will delve into the essentials of understanding nutrition, practicing portion control and mindful eating, meal planning and preparation, and making wise choices when it comes to healthy snacking.

(a) Understanding nutrition

To build healthy eating habits, it's crucial to have a fundamental understanding of nutrition. Here's what you need to know:

- **Macronutrients**: These are nutrients your body needs in larger quantities to remain healthy.

- **Micronutrients**: These are vitamins and minerals needed by the body in small amounts. Ensure your diet includes a variety of fruits, vegetables, and whole grains to get a broad spectrum of micronutrients.

- **Hydration**: Don't overlook the importance of water. Proper hydration is vital for metabolism and overall health.

- **Dietary Fiber:** Fiber is essential for digestive health and can help control hunger. Include fiber-rich foods such as grains and vegetables in your diet.

v. **Food Labels:** Pay attention to food labels and make informed choices about the nutritional content of packaged foods.

(b) Portion Control and Mindful Eating

Effective portion control and mindful eating can prevent overeating and help you develop a healthier relationship with food. Consider these strategies:

- **Serving sizes:** Understand recommended serving sizes and use measuring tools to help you become aware of portion sizes.

- **Eating Environment:** Create a calm, distraction-free eating environment. Avoid eating in front of the TV or computer to stay attuned to your body's signals of fullness.

- **Emotional Eating:** It is important to strike a balance between bodily hunger and passionate hunger. Avoid resolving to eat food when facing stress or negative emotions; rather, look out for other ways to deal with stress.

(c) Meal Planning and Preparation

Meal planning and preparation are vital tools for maintaining a healthy diet. Below are the steps for meal planning and preparation:

- **Plan Ahead:** Plan your meals for the week, including breakfast, lunch, and dinner. This eliminates the chance of unhealthy choices.
- **Grocery Shopping**: Create a shopping list in line with your meal plan. Stick to the list to avoid purchasing unnecessary, unhealthy items.

- **Batch Cooking:** Cook in batches and prepare meals in advance. This can save time and make it easier to stick to your plan during busy days.
- **Balanced Meals**: Aim for balanced meals that include a source of protein, healthy fats, and a variety of vegetables and fruits.

v. **Healthy Cooking Techniques**: Learn how to cook using healthier methods like grilling, steaming, or baking rather than frying.

(d) Healthy snacking

Healthy snacking can help maintain your energy levels and prevent overindulging during main meals. Consider these tips:

- **Snack choices**: Go for nutritious snacks like fresh fruits and vegetables with hummus, Greek yogurt, or nuts, rather than processed or sugary options.
- **Portion size**: Control your portions when snacking. Get a small container or portion of your snacks in advance.
- **Snack schedule**: Plan your snacks to coincide with your hunger levels between meals.

- **Hydration**: Sometimes, what we perceive as hunger is thirst. Drink water before reaching for a snack to see if you're genuinely hungry.

- **Avoid mindless snacking:** Avoid snacking while doing other activities, like watching TV. Instead, take a break to fully enjoy your snack.

(e) Sleeping sufficiently

Getting enough sleep is essential to maintaining a healthy weight. The hormone balance in the body can be upset by getting too little sleep which raises ghrelin (the hunger hormone) and lowers leptin (the hormone that helps you feel full).

The result of this hormone imbalance might be weight gain and overeating. Moreover, not getting enough sleep might affect your self-control and decision-making. When planning a restful sleep Schedule, take into consideration the following advice to enhance your attempts to manage your weight and encourage better sleep:

- **Regular sleep schedule**: Maintaining consistency improves the quality of your sleep by balancing your body's internal clock. Create a resting bedtime practice to let your body know when to rest.

This may involve deep breathing techniques or engaging in light physical exercise, like stretching.

- **Create a sleep-friendly Environment:** Ensure your bedroom is calm, dark, and cozy. Make your pillow and mattress are cozy. Cut Down on Screen Time: Before going to bed, stay away from devices (computers, TVs, phones, tablets), as the blue light from them can disrupt your sleep cycle. Recall your diet. Steer clear of alcohol, caffeine, and large meals right before bed.

- **Frequent Exercise**: Get moving frequently, but aim to wrap up your workouts a few hours before going to bed.

- **Treating Sleep Disorders**: You should think about seeing a medical expert if you have problems falling asleep.

Chapter 3

Designing An Effective Exercise Routine

In your weight loss journey, creating an effective exercise routine is essential for achieving your goals and improving your overall health.

The benefits of regular physical activity

Before diving into the specifics of your exercise routine, it's important to understand why regular physical activity is crucial.

- **Weight Management**: Regular exercise helps create a calorie deficit, aiding in weight loss and maintenance.

Improved Cardiovascular Health: Physical activity strengthens the heart, lowers blood pressure, and reduces the risk of heart disease.

Enhanced Metabolism: Exercise increases your resting metabolic rate, helping you burn more calories even at rest.

Muscle Strength: Strength training builds lean muscle mass, which can boost metabolism and support a toned appearance.

Better Mood: Exercise releases endorphins, which can reduce stress and anxiety while improving mood.

- **Increased Energy:** Regular physical activity enhances overall stamina and energy levels.
- **Better Sleep**: Improved sleep quality is a common benefit of exercise.
- **Enhanced Mobility**: Regular movement helps maintain joint flexibility and overall mobility.

Types of Exercises

To design an effective exercise routine, you should include a variety of exercises that target different aspects of physical fitness. Here are two fundamental types of exercises to consider:

Cardiovascular Exercise

These exercises focus on elevating your heart rate and increasing your breathing rate. These activities improve endurance and burn calories. Common forms of cardiovascular exercise include:

- Walking is a footwork exercise suitable for all fitness levels.
- Running or jogging is more intense than walking and great for calorie burn.
- Cycling is an excellent option for both indoor and outdoor exercise.
- Swimming is an exercise that requires the use of the entire body to move through water.
-

- Swimming helps to build strength, lose weight, burn calories, and relieve stress.
- Dancing is a fun way to improve your heart and lungs and increase muscular strength, endurance, and general fitness. It is an exercise for all ages, shapes, and sizes.
- Aerobics Classes: Group classes that combine music and movement for a cardio workout.
- HIIT (High-Intensity Interval Training): Short bursts of intense exercise followed by brief rest periods
- Jump Rope: An affordable and highly effective cardiovascular workout

Strength Training

Strength training, or resistance training, focuses on building and toning muscle. Incorporating this type of exercise into your routine can lead to a leaner and more sculpted physique. Key aspects of strength training include:

- Free Weights: Dumbbells, barbells, and kettlebells are effective tools for building strength.
- Bodyweight Exercises: Exercises like push-ups, squats, and planks use your body's weight for resistance.

- Resistance Bands: These provide variable resistance and are suitable for all fitness levels.
- Machines: Many gyms offer strength training machines designed to target specific muscle groups.
- Functional Training: Exercises that mimic real-life movements, such as kettlebell swings and medicine ball exercises.
- Core Work: Focusing on the core muscles with exercises like sit-ups, leg raises, and planks.
-

When designing your exercise routine, aim for a balanced combination of cardiovascular and strength-training exercises. This combination will help you burn calories, improve your cardiovascular fitness, and build muscle, all are essential for effective weight management and overall health.

Chapter 4

Managing Stress and Emotional Eating

In the journey toward weight management and overall well-being, managing stress and addressing emotional eating are critical components. This chapter explores the connection between stress and obesity, stress-reduction techniques, and strategies for coping with emotional eating.

Identifying the connection between stress and obesity

Stress and obesity often share a close relationship.

Stress can trigger obesity and make it more difficult to control. Here's how the two are connected:

- Hormonal changes: Stress triggers the release of hormones like cortisol, which can lead to increased appetite and cravings for high-calorie, sugary foods.

- Emotional eating: People always resolve to eat foods when they are stressed, leading to overeating of unhealthy diets.

- Poor sleep: Stress can disrupt sleep patterns, which can, in turn, disrupt hormonal regulation and appetite control.

- Lack of physical activity: Chronic stress can sap motivation and energy, making it more difficult to maintain an active lifestyle.

How to reduce stress

Reducing stress is crucial for both your mental and physical well-being. Below are the techniques for stress-reduction:

- Mindfulness meditation: Practice mindfulness to stay in the present moment, reducing anxiety and stress levels.
- Deep breathing: Engage in deep, diaphragmatic breathing to calm your nervous system and reduce stress.

- Yoga: Regular yoga sessions can help alleviate stress, improve flexibility, and enhance mental clarity.

- Engage in physical activities to reduce stress and improve mood.

- Progressive muscle relaxation: Learn to release muscle tension systematically, promoting relaxation.

- Time management: Organize your tasks and set achievable goals to prevent overstressing yourself.

- Social support: Talk to friends and family or consider joining a support group to share your experiences and seek advice.

- Hobbies: Engage in physical activities you enjoy doing to relax and keep your mind happy.

Handling with emotional eating

Emotional eating often arises when reacting to negative or positive emotions. When battling with emotional eating, it is important to know when you are eating to feel satisfied or to relieve stress. This can help to stop emotional and stressful eating, fight cravings, and find more satisfying ways to feed your feelings. Below are some tips to be considered when dealing with emotional eating:

- Awareness: Keep abreast of the things that trigger emotional eating. Keep a diary to identify trends.
- Alternative coping strategies: Find non-food-related ways to manage stress and emotions, such as exercise, meditation, or talking to a friend.
- Mindful eating: Practice mindful eating by paying attention to what and why you eat. If you observe that you often eat for boredom or comfort, you may be eating for emotional reasons.

- Keep Healthy Snacks Available: Stock your kitchen with nutritious options to minimize the availability of unhealthy comfort foods.
- Control Portion: If you do eat emotionally, use a smaller plate to prevent overloading.
- Determine Triggers: Determine the circumstances or feelings that lead to your emotional eating.
- Look for substitutes: Create more constructive coping mechanisms for your emotions, such as going for a stroll, talking to a friend, or engaging in a pastime.

- Maintain a food journal: Monitoring your consumption of food might assist you in recognizing emotional eating behaviors.

- Eating with awareness: Consider what you're eating and why. Refrain from eating out of boredom or habit.

- Seek Professional Assistance: Seeking support from a therapist or counselor is a good idea if emotional eating is a recurring issue.

Chapter 5

Seeking Support and Accountability,

Establishing a Support Network: A strong support system is essential for managing weight in an efficient manner. Friends, family, or medical experts can offer emotional support, motivation, and direction along your trip.

Getting Involved in Weight Loss Communities and Groups: Engaging in online discussion boards or support groups for weight loss can result in enlightening exchanges, motivation, and practical advice.

You can stay accountable by learning from people who have similar goals to yours and by sharing experiences with them.

Tracking Your Progress: It is vital to monitor your progress, including your weight, dietary decisions, and exercise routines, to identify trends and identify areas that require improvement. Keeping a journal of your achievements will support your motivation.

Maintaining your achievements

Sustaining your weight loss is just as important as achieving it.

It involves maintaining a healthy lifestyle and preventing weight regain by adhering to the step-by-step produces to achieve your desired goal.

Handling plateau in weight loss

Plateaus in weight loss are common and can be annoying. To get over them, think about changing your diet or exercise regimen, getting advice from medical professionals, and keeping in mind the progress you've previously accomplished. Here are some methods for breaking past a weight reduction plateau:

- Reassess your objectives: Examine your weight loss objectives more closely. Are they feasible, long-term, and healthy?

If your expectations are overly ambitious, it may be time to lower them.

- Examine your diet: Examine your existing eating patterns. Are you accurately tracking your calorie intake? To generate a calorie deficit, make sure you consume less calories than you burn.

- Change up your diet: Consider adjusting your diet if you've been following one. Your body may have been accustomed to your existing eating habits. To jumpstart your metabolism, experiment with different foods or meal plans.

- Portion size control: Keep portion proportions in mind and try not to overeat. Smaller and more balanced meals can help you control your calorie intake and avoid overindulging.

Increase the variety of your meals by doing the following:

- Include a variety of items in your diet to ensure you obtain a variety of nutrients. This can help keep your metabolism active and minimize boredom.
- Increase your protein consumption: Protein can help you feel full while also preserving muscle mass.

Consider including additional lean protein sources in your diet.

- Keep hydrated: Water consumption is critical for weight loss. Your body may occasionally confuse thirst with hunger, leading to overeating. Throughout the day, drink lots of water.

- Change the macronutrient ratios: Experiment with various macronutrient ratios, such as decreasing carbohydrates while increasing healthy fats and proteins.

- Increase your physical activity level: Incorporate or up the amount of physical activity in your routine if you're not already.

To increase your metabolism and burn more calories, combine weight training with cardiovascular exercise.

- Modify your exercise regimen: Your body may adjust to your workout regimen, producing less noticeable effects. To challenge your muscles and metabolism, try new exercises, up the intensity, or alter your training routine.

- Observe how stressed you are: Excessive stress might impede weight loss or cause weight gain. Use stress-reduction strategies, including yoga, meditation, and mindfulness.

- Make sleep a priority: Make sure you're receiving plenty of restful sleep. Hormone control can be upset by sleep deprivation, which makes weight loss more difficult.

- Follow your development: Maintain a thorough journal of your meals, workouts, and other activities that affect your ability to lose weight. Finding trends or potential improvement areas can be aided by this data.

- Speak with a medical professional: Should you find yourself stuck on a plateau, you might want to speak with a qualified dietician or other healthcare professional.

They can handle any underlying medical concerns and offer tailored advice.

- Remain persistent and patient: If you stick with your diet and goals, plateaus are a natural aspect of losing weight and will eventually pass. Remain persistent and don't give up.

It may require some time and work to break through a weight loss plateau, but with the correct modifications and perseverance, you can keep moving in the direction of your weight reduction objectives.

Health and safety considerations

While a step-by-step obesity treatment plan can be helpful, it is critical to prioritize your health and safety throughout the process.

Consult your medical professional
Consult with your healthcare professional before beginning any serious weight loss journey, especially if you have underlying medical concerns.

Avoid excessive diets: Extreme diets can be dangerous. Always choose a long-term strategy that promotes health.

Keep hydrated: Adequate water consumption is essential for body processes and general health.

Be Conscious of Your Body: Pay keen attention to your body's cues. If you are feeling ill or too tired, it is critical that you take a step back and rethink your strategy.

Psychological Planning

Rapid weight loss necessitates both physical and mental effort. A positive mindset is essential for success. Consider the following psychological strategies:

Positive Self-Talk: Be gentle with yourself and use positive self-talk.

Believe in your ability to achieve your objectives.

Visualize Success: Visualization techniques can be extremely effective. Consider how you will feel when you reach your goal weight.

Managing Stress: Managing stress is important since it can lead to emotional eating. Consider incorporating stress-reduction practices into your routine, such as meditation, deep breathing, or yoga.

Accountability means holding yourself responsible for your actions.

Review your progress on a regular basis and make improvements as appropriate.

Managing medical intervention

When to Think About Getting Medical Help: When traditional weight-loss techniques fail, medical intervention might be required, particularly if you have health problems associated with obesity. To find out if medical intervention is the best course of action, speak with a healthcare professional.

Medical treatment types

Examine the various medical interventions that can help with weight management.

a.   **Prescription drugs**: By reducing hunger or altering how your body breaks down food, several drugs can aid in weight loss.

b.   **Bariatric surgery**: When other approaches have failed to produce noticeable weight loss, surgical procedures such as gastric bypass or gastric sleeve surgery may be useful.

Conclusion

"Step by Step Obesity Remedy: A Complete Guide to Overcoming Obesity and Living a Healthier Life" provides readers with a well-structured and educational way to deal with the essential issue of obesity. This guide takes a comprehensive approach to addressing the numerous difficulties of obesity, emphasizing that sustainable change is attainable with education, determination, and a commitment to a healthier lifestyle.

We have discussed numerous elements of obesity throughout the book, from understanding its causes and implications to implementing practical weight-management measures.

The step-by-step method gives clarity and advice, allowing readers to progress at their own pace and making it accessible to anybody looking to live a better life. This book emphasizes the significance of laying a strong foundation for health through nutrition, exercise, stress management, and emotional well-being. It inspires readers to take charge of their lives and make decisions that will benefit their long-term health and well-being.

The chapters on support and accountability, and overcoming plateaus remind us that the route to a better life is not without hurdles, but barriers may be conquered with perseverance and the correct tools.

It emphasizes the need to receive help from friends, family, and communities, as well as the need for an internal drive to keep going. Furthermore, the discussion of medical therapies and long-term maintenance serves as a reminder that there are other paths to success in obesity remedy. It encourages readers to seek professional assistance as necessary, and they must remain watchful to maintain their gains.

As we come to the end of this thorough book, keep in mind that the journey to a better life is an ongoing one.

By putting the principles and tactics presented in this book into action, you will have the knowledge and resources you need to conquer obesity and embark on a lifelong path to better health, well-being, and a brighter, more vibrant future. Your dedication to living a healthier lifestyle is admirable, and with the knowledge obtained from this guide, you are well-prepared to confront the obstacles and celebrate the victories that lie ahead.